THE BEST FOOD ON THE PLANET TO HELP YOU CONCEIVE AND WHY

Written By: Sam Hall

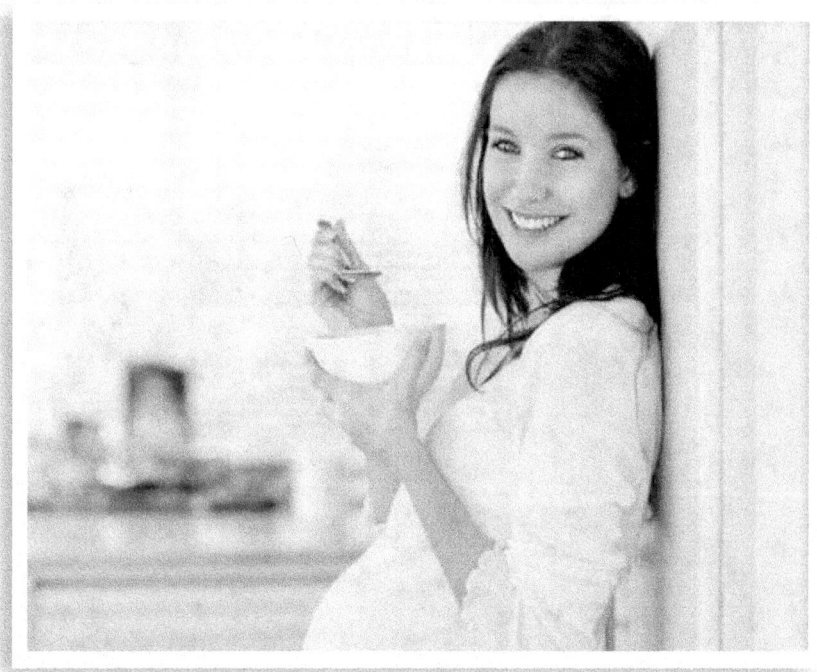

Becoming a mother is a main priority for many women, and the journey to conception can be time consuming and frustrating. In preparation for all of the restrictions you are about to experience once baby is in your belly, why not maximize your chances of conception by incorporating food into your diet that are proven to prime the rails?

PAY ATTENTION TO YOUR PROTEINS

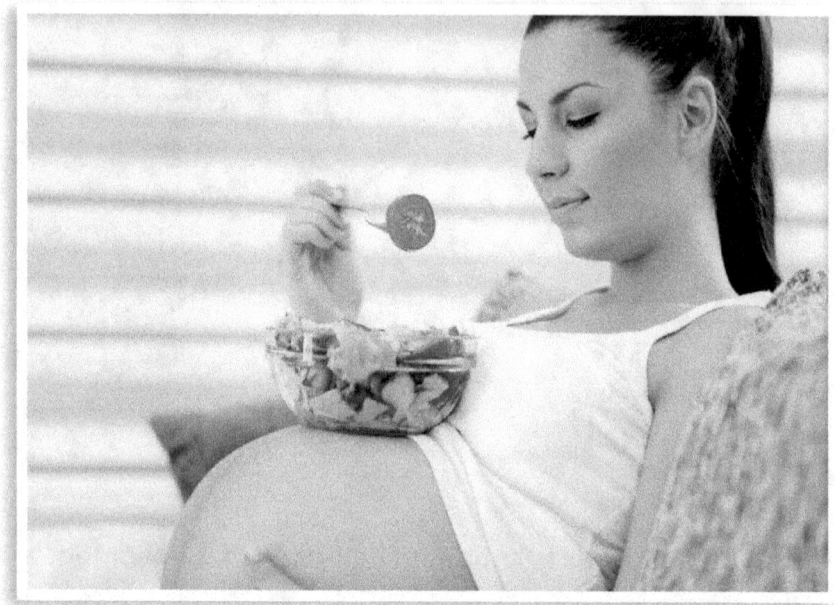

A Harvard study indicated that women who consume mostly animal proteins were more likely to have trouble conceiving than women who consumed more plant proteins. So bring on the lentils, tofu, beans, edamame, and nuts!

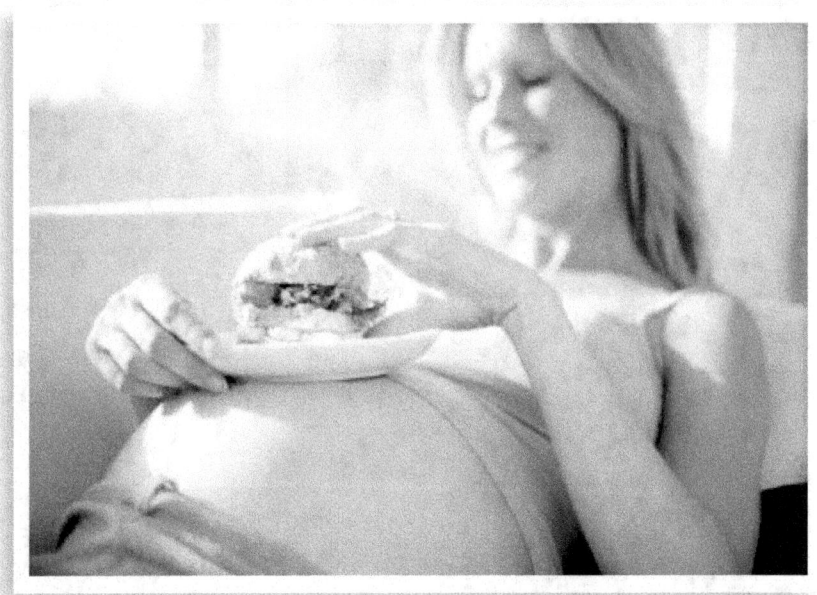

If raw and whole plant proteins are not your thing, try to find a good veggie burger to pop on the grill. Find a great vegetarian chili recipe, and buy yourself a vegan cookbook or two. No one is saying you need to cut out the steaks altogether, but diversified protein sources are the name of your preconception game!

GET SOME WHOLE DAIRY

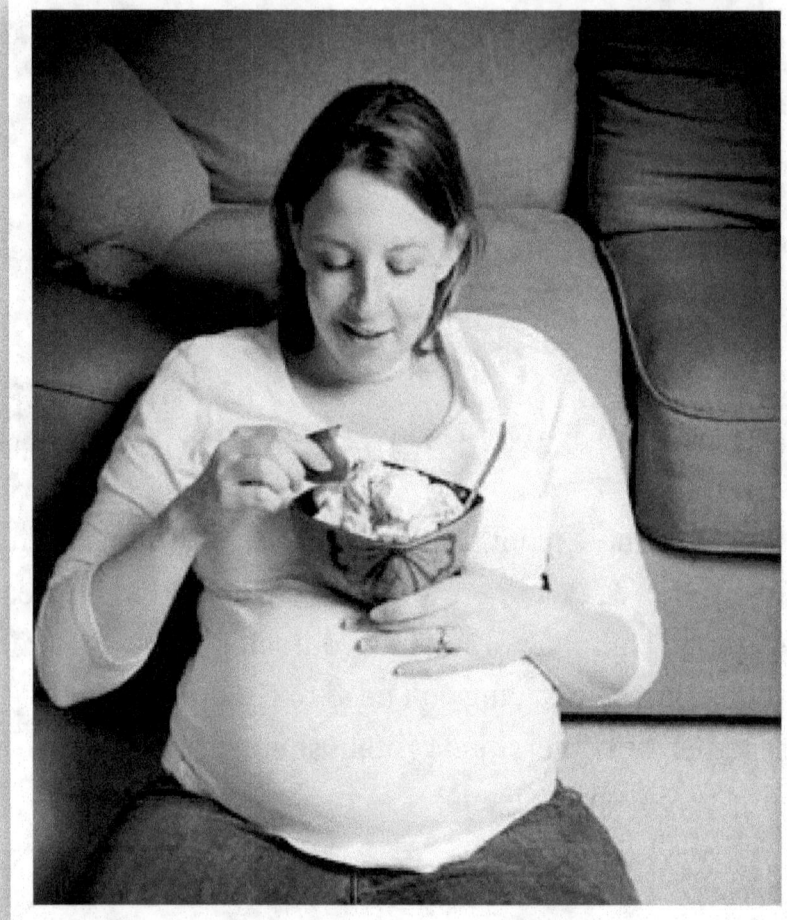

The verdict is in: your little eggs love themselves some whole-fat dairy. Bring on the (real) ice cream and whole milk! One serving a day will usually do it, unless you're working hard in other areas to maintain a healthy prepregnancy weight.

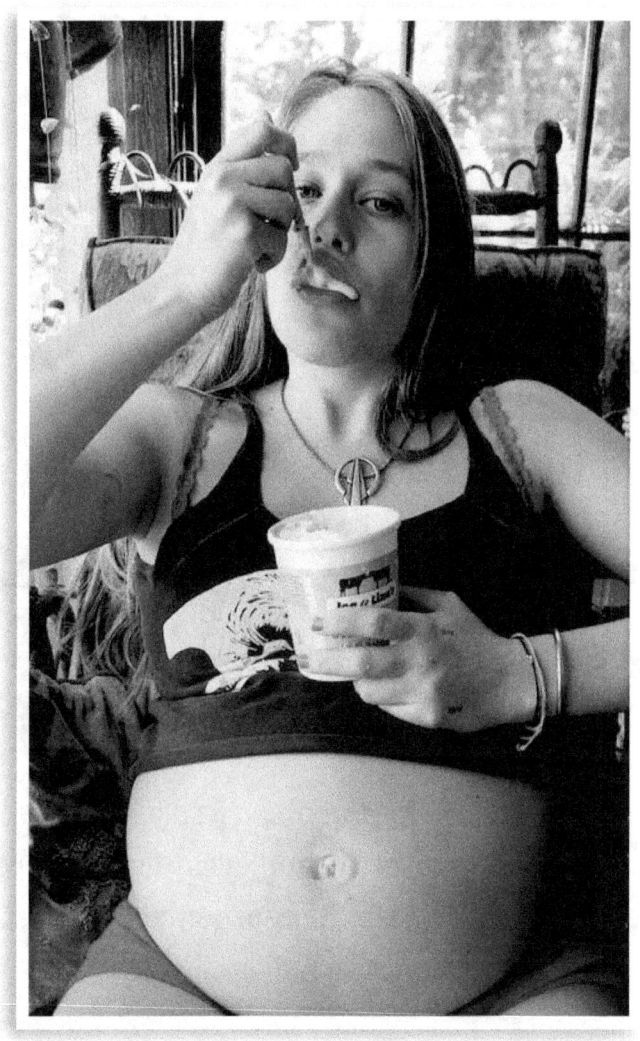

The reasons for this added benefit are a mystery, though some say the removal of fat from milk actually messes with the hormonal balance, which can have a negative effect on your own hormones. As an added bonus, you'll be packing in some extra calcium, which will fortify your soon to be depleted reserves.

WATCH YOUR FISH!

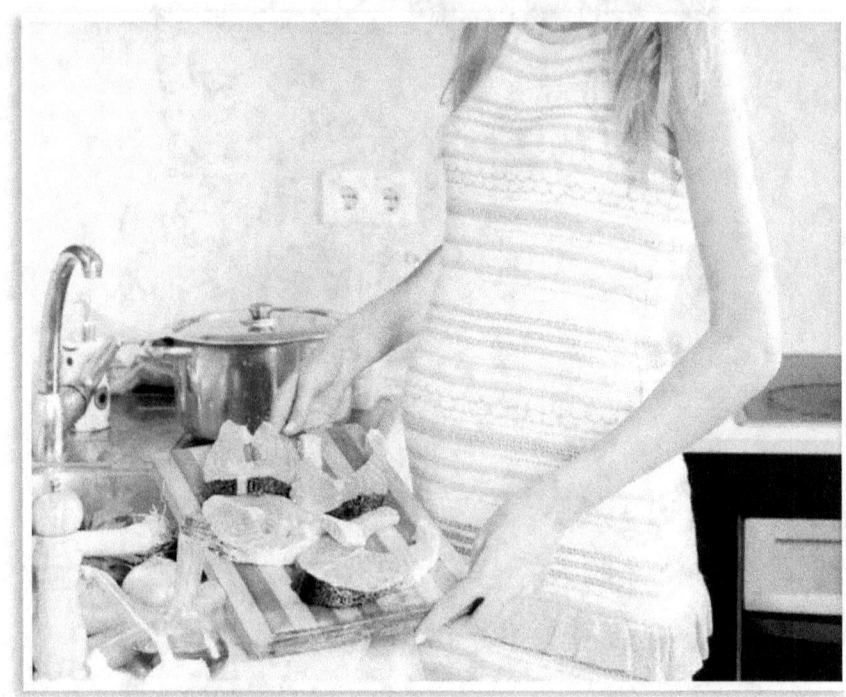

Fish itself is beneficial for the omega-3s which aid in healthy development of brain and eyes. Pre conception, it increases the blood flow to the reproductive organs and may even boost reproductive hormones.

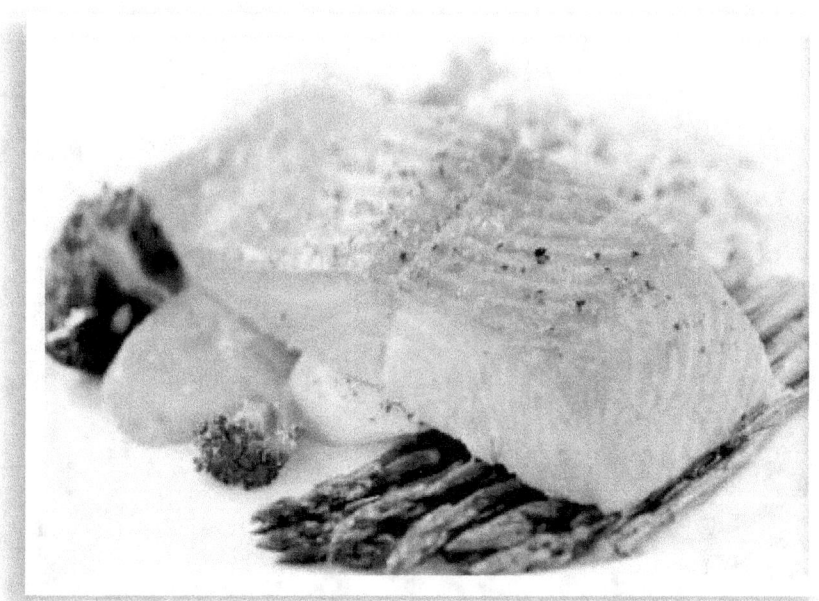

Wild salmon makes the must eat list because it is lower in mercury than most other fish on the market. It's also available in forms other than filets, like prepackaged salmon burgers. It's recommended that women who are trying to conceive avoid swordfish, tilefish, and mackerel, so make sure you do some research before you branch into exotic waters.

SWAP YOUR OILS

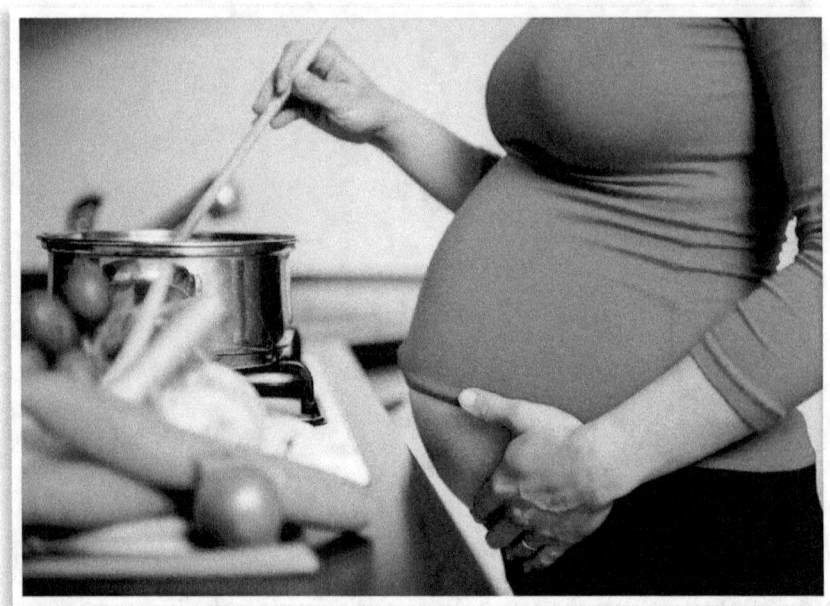

While vegetable oils are more economical, there are some definite benefits to switching over to olive oil. Besides, olive oil just tastes better anyway, so fork over the extra coin and get something that will help you build your family while tasting great!

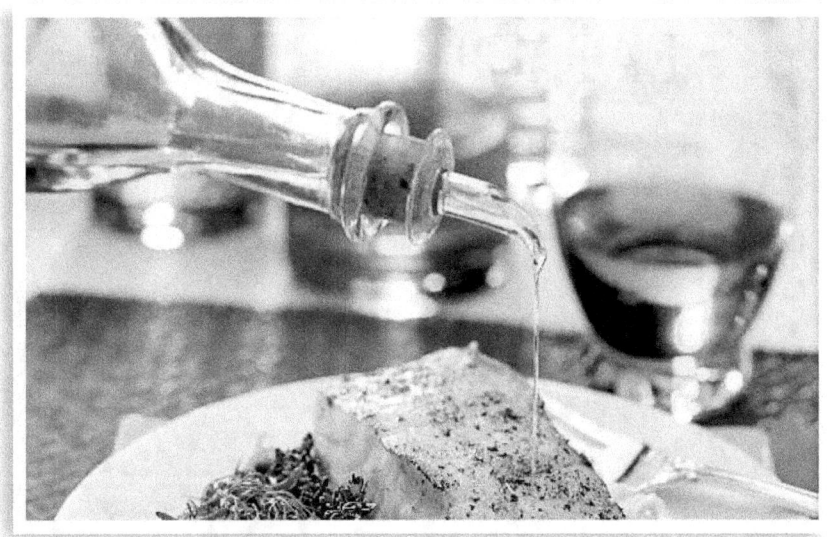

Olive oil is a monounsaturated fat, which is another way of saying that it does your pre-pregnancy body good. It is proven to reduce inflammation, which is a major hinderance to conception.

EAT YOUR GREENS!

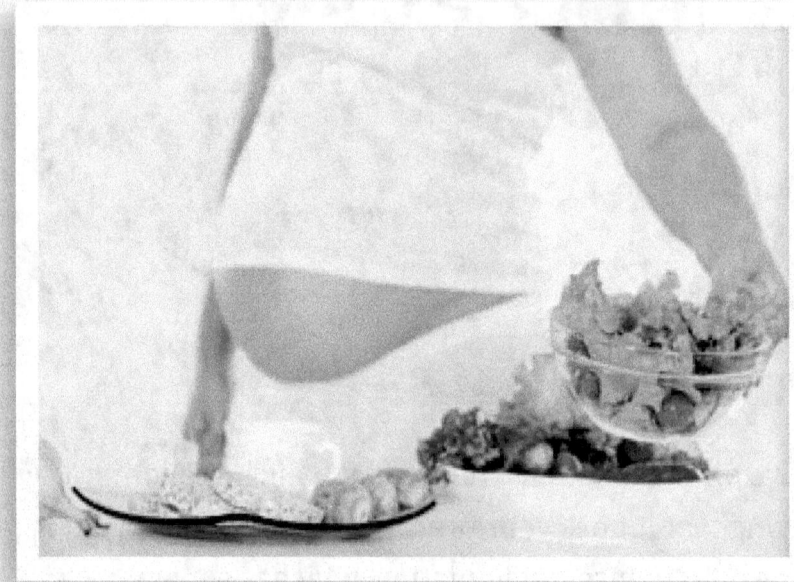

Folate is a key nutrient for the health of your future infant. Eating foods high in this nutrient, as well as taking a folic acid supplement, can prepare your body for a healthy pregnancy. Leafy greens, such as kale, romaine, spinach, arugula, and broccoli, are all great sources and should form a large part of your pre-pregnancy diet.

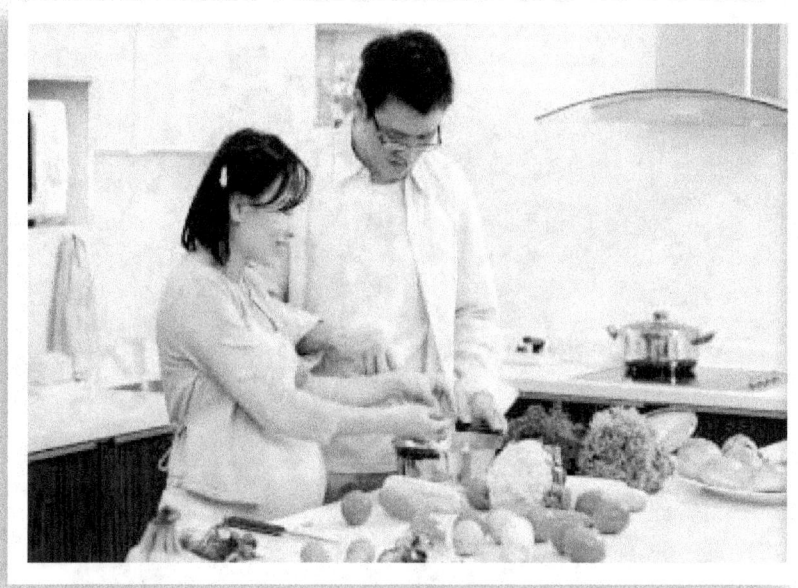

It's even been proven that men who have diet high in folate have healthier sperm overall, so get your partner in on the game plan. Not that you have to eat salad exclusively. There are plenty of ways to incorporate greens into your diet, so try some soups and lettuce wraps to make things interesting.

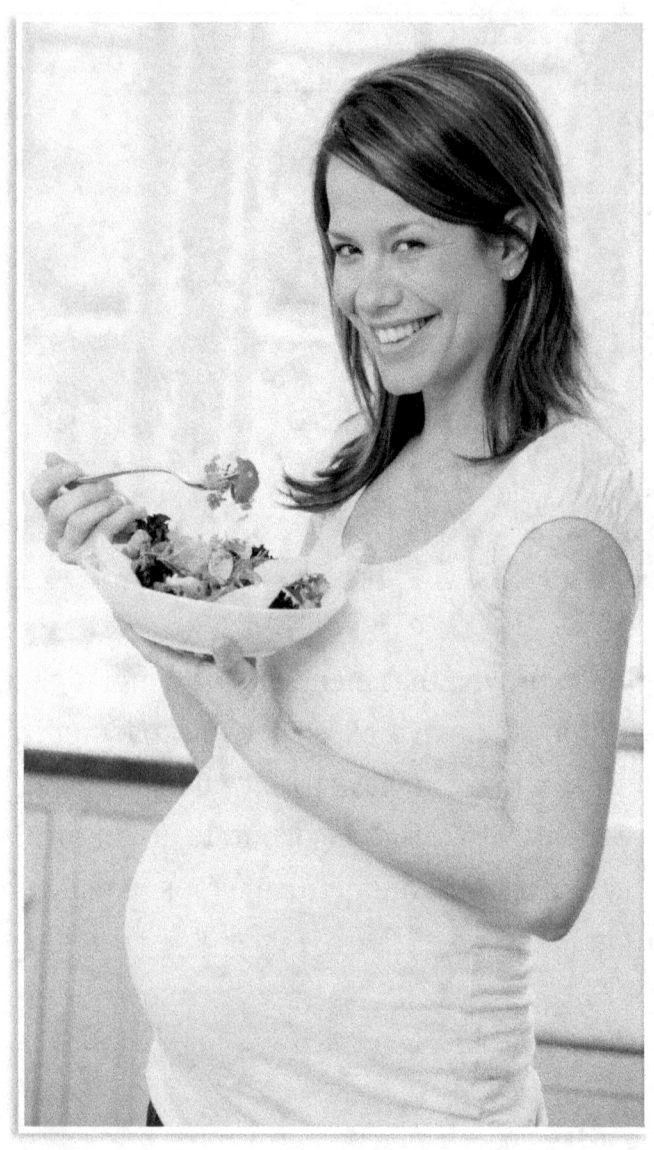

The benefits of folate are no joke for your future babes. High consumption of this nutrient is linked to a lower risk of miscarriage and healthier cardiovascular systems.

GET SOME IRON

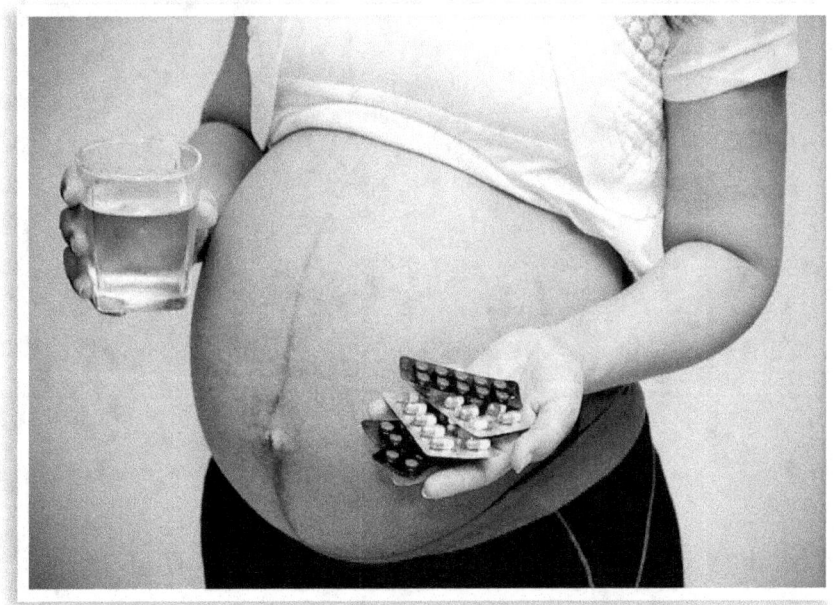

In one study, women who regularly took an iron supplement were 40% less likely to have trouble with conception! Then again, if you're already popping a prenatal vitamin you've probably had your fill of supplements in pill form.

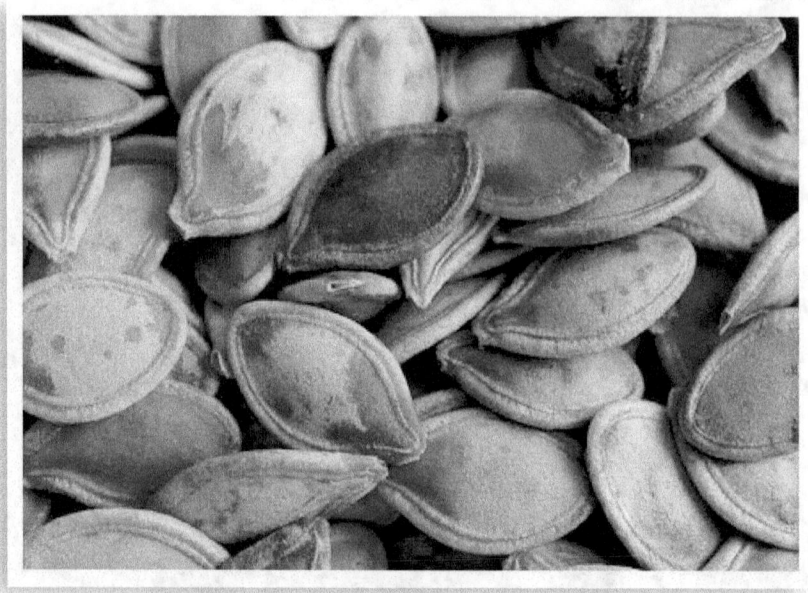

Instead of grabbing yet another pill in the pharmacy section, toast some pumpkin seeds which are high in heme iron. This is the type of iron that is the most easily absorbed and beneficial to the body. You'll also benefit from having this crunchy snack on hand when the craving for potato chips and pretzels hits you.

WHOLE GRAINS

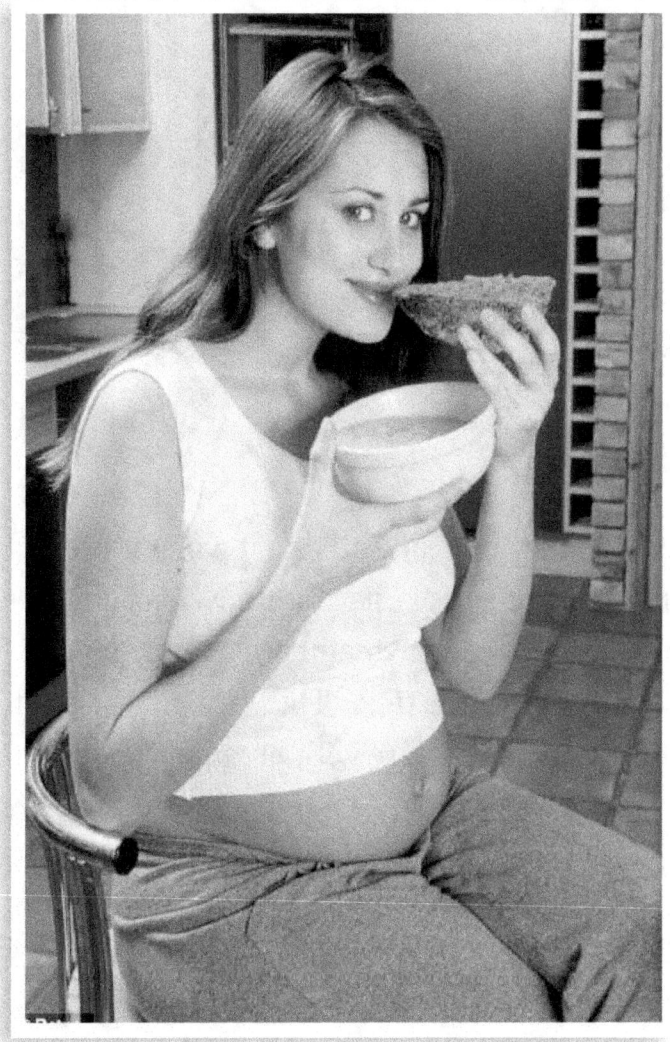

As a general rule, dark breads with whole grains are slower to digest. These help you maintain your blood sugar levels, avoiding potentially harmful spikes and valleys.

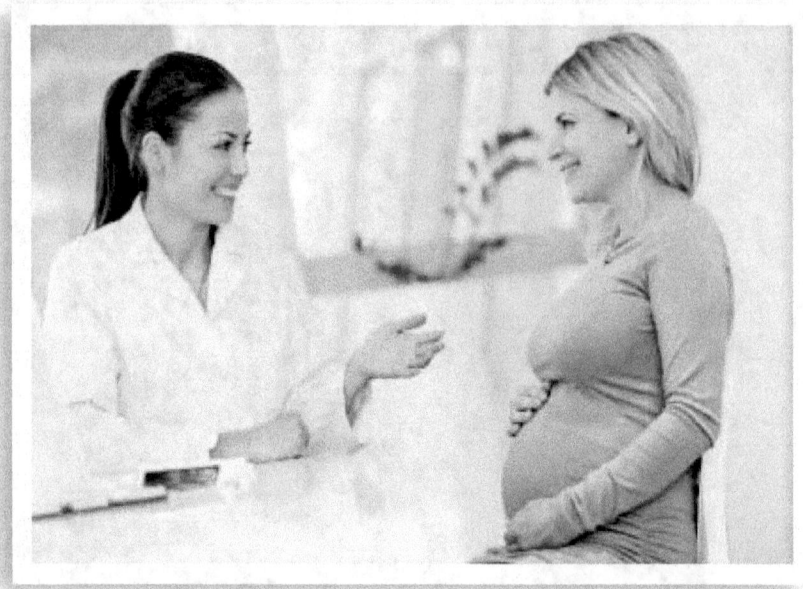

A study out of Europe indicated that women whose blood sugar ran high had a 60% harder time conceiving over 6 months than women who maintained lower levels of blood sugar consistently over time. This is because higher levels of insulin actually interfere with pregnancy hormones.

CUT OUT BAD FAT

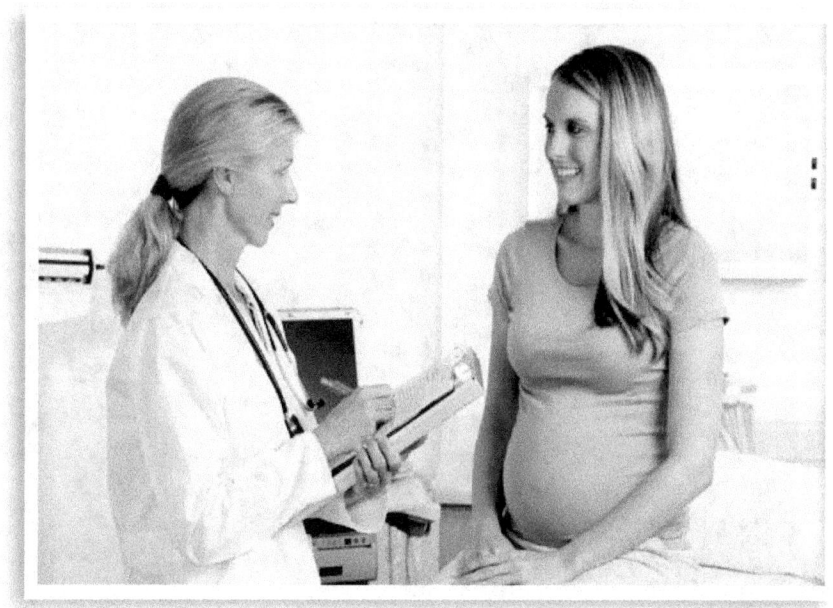

Trans fats, which are found in many fried and processed foods, are a no-go when it comes to trying to conceive. These delicious, delicious gremlins can interfere with your hormones to the point of causing irregular ovulation!

GET YOUR VITAMIN C

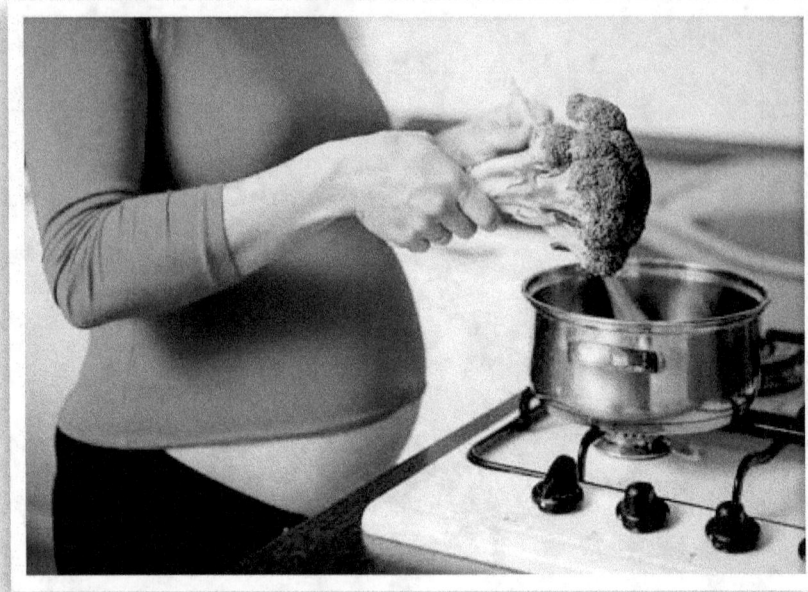

Foods high in vitamin C, such as bell peppers and broccoli, can help you to absorb all of that extra iron you're consuming for the benefit of your future little one. It will also fortify your immune system against those sneaky seasonal colds that can put you down for the count.

CUT OUT ALCOHOL

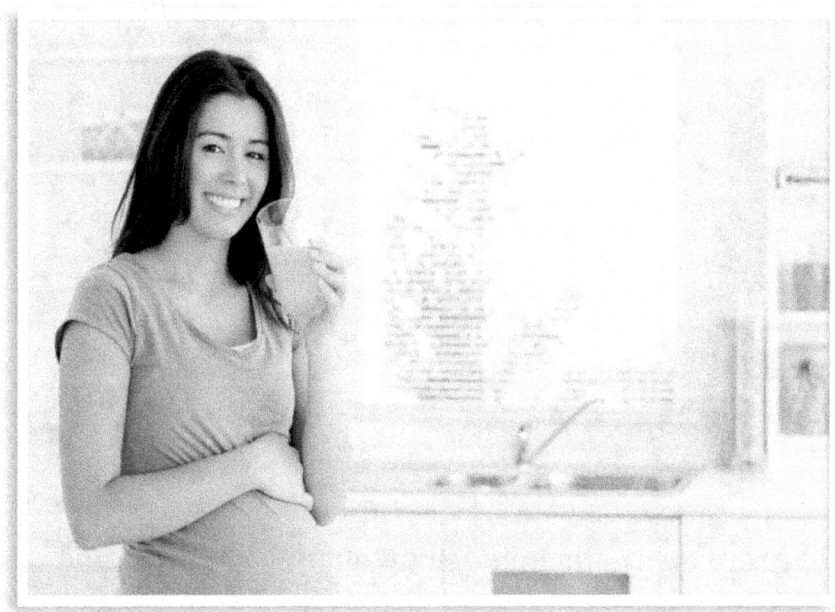

Ok, it seems like this may be putting the cart before the horse as you're likely looking at well over 9 months with no delicious booze anyway. Hear me out: multiple studies have shown that even moderate alcohol consumption can interfere with conception. So, perhaps find another way to prime yourself for some lovin rather than that glass of red wine.

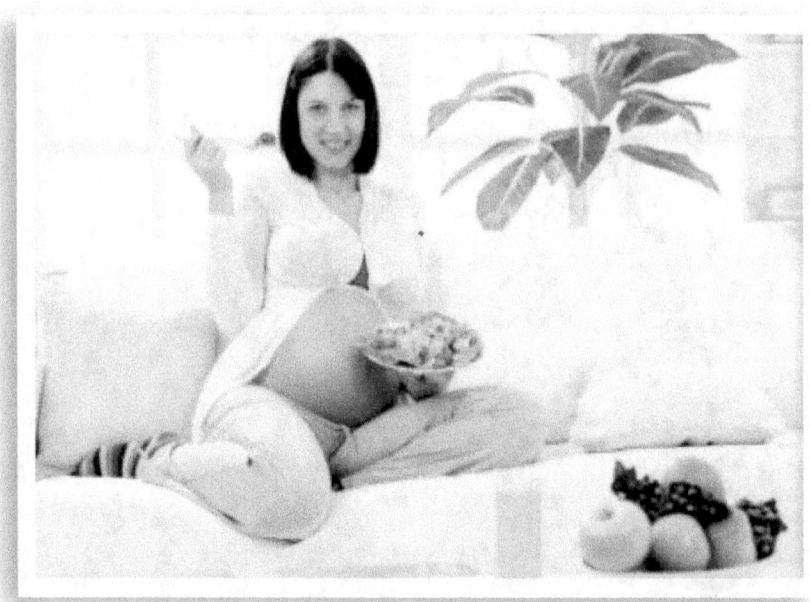

There are many other guidelines about what to eat and when, but incorporate these principles into your food routine and you'll be priming your body for optimal performance and a healthy pregnancy.

Thank You!

We hope you enjoyed the book! All pictures and words were lovingly put together by experts who really love what they do! We really hope you learned something new today!

We would really appreciate it, if you could PLEASE take the time to let us know how we're doing by leaving a review on the Amazon website. We appreciate any comments you may have – what you enjoyed about the book, what additions you would have liked to have seen and what you would like to see in future publications.

Any comments will help understand better what you and your kids most enjoy and allows us to better provide exactly what you want!

Thought Junction Publishing

A NOTE FROM THE WRITER

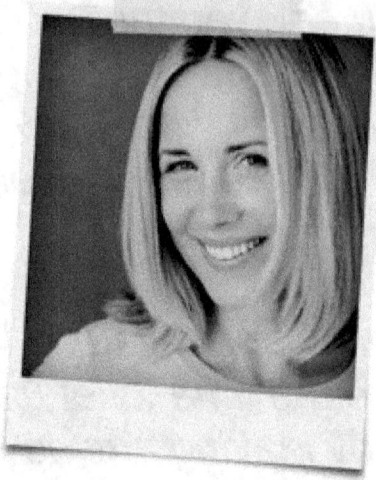

Sam's life revolves around her family, devoted mother of 3 - Noah (6), Oscar (3) and Poppy (11months) - she writes in a real way, aiming to answer the questions that other books don't cover, to fill in the blanks and inform parents and parents-to-be of the truth about raising children in the modern world.

Sam's writings emphasize that the readers are not alone - that there is a community of support available, and other people to talk to who can help, support and assist.

When she's not writing books, Sam is an advisor and avid blogger for Ideal Parent - http://ideal-parent.com - spreading support, care and advice across the web!

Join Sam on Ideal Parent and keep an eye out for her books - she's on a mission to help parents worldwide - join her and spread the word!